Francisco Marques
Catarina Lopes
Magda Guerra

FUNCTIONAL INDEPENDENCE OF THE POST-STROKE PATIENT

Francisco Marques
Catarina Lopes
Magda Guerra

FUNCTIONAL INDEPENDENCE OF THE POST-STROKE PATIENT

Importance of the rehabilitation program

ScienciaScripts

Imprint
Any brand names and product names mentioned in this book are subject to trademark, brand or patent protection and are trademarks or registered trademarks of their respective holders. The use of brand names, product names, common names, trade names, product descriptions etc. even without a particular marking in this work is in no way to be construed to mean that such names may be regarded as unrestricted in respect of trademark and brand protection legislation and could thus be used by anyone.

Cover image: www.ingimage.com

This book is a translation from the original published under ISBN 978-620-6-76085-6.

Publisher:
Sciencia Scripts
is a trademark of
Dodo Books Indian Ocean Ltd. and OmniScriptum S.R.L publishing group

120 High Road, East Finchley, London, N2 9ED, United Kingdom
Str. Armeneasca 28/1, office 1, Chisinau MD-2012, Republic of Moldova, Europe
Printed at: see last page
ISBN: 978-620-8-13667-3

FUNCTIONAL INDEPENDENCE OF THE POST-STROKE PATIENT

THINKING

"The brain is an enchanted loom where millions of glowing shuttles (nerve impulses) weave a scattered pattern, a pattern always full of meaning and yet never lasting; a harmony of constantly changing sub-patterns. "

Charles Sherington

ACKNOWLEDGEMENTS

This study received important support and incentives without which it would not have become a reality.

To relatives, colleagues and stroke victims,

To everyone, our recognition and gratitude!

SUMMARY

Introduction: According to Neri (2001), functional capacity/independence has been defined as the degree of preservation of the individual's ability to carry out basic activities of daily living (BADLs) or self-care and also to develop instrumental activities of daily living (IADLs). Stroke is, for all intents and purposes, the manifestation of a cerebral vascular disease, and its consequences are varied and depend on the extent and location of the nerve tissue damage (Cambier *et al,* 2005). The aim of the rehabilitation process is to minimise the impact of the stroke on both the victim and their carer. Given this framework, the research aimed to identify levels of functional independence in post-stroke patients and their correlation with sociodemographic and clinical variables, comparing functional independence on admission with discharge.

Methods: A cross-sectional, analytical-correlational, quantitative, descriptive study was carried out in which 60 patients, mostly male (60%) and with an average age of 60.8 years, were admitted to the Alcoitão Rehabilitation Medicine Centre. Data collection included a sociodemographic characterisation questionnaire, a clinical characterisation questionnaire and the Functional Independence Measure Scale (FIM).

Results: The evidence found in this study shows that functional independence had an increase in all dimensions of the Functional Independence Measurement Scale (FIM) when comparing the time of entry with that of discharge. The variables that significantly influenced functional independence were marital status (self-care dimension), stroke duration (self-care, sphincter and locomotion dimensions), rehabilitation in the acute phase (self-care, locomotion and mobility dimensions) and the ongoing rehabilitation programme.

Conclusion: Clinical variables have a greater influence on functional independence when tested dimension by dimension. In view of the above, we can conclude that the rehabilitation programme plays a key role in the patient's functional independence, so it should be started as early as possible and continued energetically.

Key words: Patient, Post Stroke, Functional Independence

INDICE

INTRODUCTION

The term Cerebral Vascular Accident (CVA) refers to a set of symptoms of neurological impairment resulting from brain lesions caused by altered blood supply (PHIPPS, 2003).

Stroke is, for all intents and purposes, the manifestation of a cerebral vascular disease, and its consequences are varied and depend on the extent and location of the nerve tissue damage (CAMBIER *et al,* 2005).

According to PORTUGAL (2009), the Portuguese population that has or has had a stroke is 17,163,38, affecting 89,293 males and 82,345 females.

Stroke is a major public health problem and is considered one of the main contributors to morbidity and mortality worldwide. According to PORTUGAL (2000), 20,995 stroke patients died in Portugal, making it one of the main causes of death. According to the *EUROPEAN STROKE ORGANISATION* (2003), in industrialised countries it is the third most frequent cause of death, after cardiovascular disease and cancer.

At the end of the 19th century and the beginning of the 20th century, stroke was seen as a fatal disease and little was known about its prevention. The only aim of rehabilitation was to maintain musculoskeletal functionality or to give the patient a peaceful death.

Studies carried out over the last few decades have led to a better understanding and the establishment of new perspectives on the problem, which has led to a considerable reduction in stroke mortality. The mortality rate has fallen by around 33 per cent since 1980, but around 25 per cent of victims are left with physical or mental disabilities that require ongoing support in life activities (PHIPPS, 2003).

The standardised mortality rate for Portugal in 2005 was 11.6%, falling in 2007 to 11.4% (PORTUGAL, 2007). Cerebrovascular disease accounts for 10% of all deaths, 9% in males and 11% in females (NOGUEIRA, 2007).

The incidence of stroke varies in different European countries, with an estimated 100 to 200 new cases/100,000 inhabitants/year. In-hospital lethality due to stroke has also been falling by around 1.9 per cent between 2004 and 2006. Although there has been no significant change in the incidence of strokes, their prevalence in the population is growing due to increased survival and the growth of the elderly population. The fact that demographic trends are moving in the direction of an ageing population will mean that the quantity and quality of specialised healthcare will be increasingly in demand (PORTUGAL, 2001).

Cerebrovascular disease is very common in the elderly, although it can affect younger age groups. Under the age of 40, it affects 3 to 5 per cent of individuals, with a higher incidence in males. However, as the age group rises, the incidence increases and the difference between the sexes narrows to very similar figures for men and women over 65.

According to FERRO (2006), there are two basic types of stroke: ischaemic and haemorrhagic. The former is caused by the occlusion of a blood vessel and can be of thrombolic or embolic origin. Thrombolic origin arises when small emboli, usually of cardiac origin, move around and become lodged in small vessels, causing a loss of blood supply. Thrombolytic strokes result from the accumulation of atheromatous plaques in the lumen of vessels.

Haemorrhagic strokes are divided into intracerebral and subarachnoid. Around 85% of strokes are ischaemic and 15% haemorrhagic.

Bearing in mind that ischaemic stroke is the most prevalent type of stroke, resulting in numerous disabilities, it became essential to find specific therapeutic solutions, with the main aim of saving the ischaemic area and minimising functional deficits. Thrombolysis was therefore used, but it has numerous inclusion criteria and many associated risks, so patient screening must be very thorough.

In a study carried out by ABREU (2009), of the 88 patients with ischaemic stroke who were admitted to the Stroke Unit of the Cova da Beira Hospital Centre, only 7.9% underwent thrombolysis. Of all the patients who underwent thrombolysis, 71.1% had a very positive response to treatment.

Despite the above, not all authors support the same idea, as TEIXEIRA (2004) stated that thrombolytic treatment was not effective in the presence of early hypodensity greater than a third of the length of the middle cerebral artery territory, and also increased the risk of intracranial haemorrhage.

Risk factors are mostly linked to behaviours and lifestyles, which change over time, and can be divided into two broad categories, modifiable and non-modifiable, as shown in the following tables.

Table 1 - Non-modifiable risk factors for stroke

Age	The risk of stroke increases with age, with 60 to 70 per cent occurring in people over 65 (PHIPPS, 2003).
Gender	The incidence is slightly higher in men (PHIPPS, 2003).
Heredity	The prevalence is four times higher when the parents also suffer from this pathology (ANDRÉ, 1999).

Table 2 - Modifiable risk factors for stroke

Hypertension	According to CHAVES (2008), hypertension is the most important modifiable risk factor, and this opinion is shared by CARMONA (2004).
Diabetes Mellitus	In the opinion of CHAVES (2008), the risk of developing a stroke in diabetics is twice as high, and this opinion is shared by André (1999). According to KOIZUMI and DICCINI (2006), treatment for diabetics and hypertensive patients should be intensified and strict blood pressure control is recommended.
Dyslipidaemia	Physical activity reduces the risk of developing a stroke, as it helps to keep cholesterol levels below 160mg/dl (André, 1999). According to CHAVES (2008), dyslipidaemia is an important risk factor for cardiovascular disease, but the relationship between serum cholesterol levels and the incidence of this disease seems to be more complex, showing that it is only a weak risk factor for ischaemic events.

Alcohol	Alcohol consumption increases the risk of haemorrhagic stroke (FERRO, 2000).
Smoking	This is the second biggest risk factor and can increase the risk up to three times (FERRO, 2000). According to CHAVES (2008), one study showed a 2.58-fold increase in the risk of cardiovascular disease in smokers compared to non-smokers, with a reduction in excess risk after quitting smoking.
Obesity	Increased body weight, especially when located in the abdominal region, is considered a cardiovascular risk factor CHAVES (2008).

SULLIVAN (1993) states that the expression of lesions caused by stroke refers to a set of signs and symptoms of neurological impairment, which are caused by altered blood supply and depend on the extent and location of the lesion in the nervous tissue and the volume of the contralateral circulation. There are physical, emotional and behavioural changes that often condition adherence to the rehabilitation programme, and it is crucial that the rehabilitation nurse always takes all these factors into account when planning and carrying out the rehabilitation process. The clinical manifestations underlying this condition include changes in function in various areas, as shown in the following table.

Chart 3 - Clinical manifestations after stroke

Motor	Hemiplegia, hemiparesis, ataxia and dysphagia
Balance	Static and dynamic standing or sitting, which occurs due to muscle weakness
Communication	Dysarthria, dysphasia or aphasia
Vision	Haemianopsia, loss of peripheral vision and diplopia
Perception	Tactile, loss of proprioception and difficulty interpreting visual and auditory stimuli
Emotional and psychological state	Loss of control, emotional lability, lower tolerance to stressful situations, isolation, fear, hostility, anger and depression
Disposal	Incontinence, bladder atony and urinary urgency
Mental activity	Decreased ability to memorise recent and long-term facts, difficulty with orientation, concentration, abstract reasoning and judgement.

PHIPPS (2003) argues that our increased knowledge of the functions of each side of the brain makes it possible to predict the effects of a stroke on each of the hemispheres. Thus, the effects of a stroke in the left hemisphere will manifest in the right hemisphere and vice versa (laterality effect), because the nerve bundles cross at the level of the brainstem (Chart 4).

Chart 4 - Left Hemisphere/Right Hemisphere Stroke

Left hemisphere stroke	Right hemisphere stroke
Motor deficits in the right hemisphere	Motor deficits in the left hemisphere
Right visual field deficits	Left visual field deficits
High level of frustration/depression over losses	Apparently unconcerned about losses
Extreme anxiety before trying new skills	Impulsiveness, highly unconcentrated
Language deficits	Perceptual-spatial deficits
Slow and cautious behaviour **Intellectual deficit**	Denial or unawareness of deficits Lack of discernment, overestimation of abilities

Source: Adap. PHIPPS [*et al]* *Medical-Surgical Nursing - Concepts and clinical practice*. 2003; 1983 p

The left hemisphere acts predominantly in the area of language, and is considered the main centre for language and calculation, control of gestural and intentional activity, especially in activities that require the participation of two-handed activities and symbolic gestures. Aphasias are characteristic of lesions in this hemisphere or the dominant hemisphere, so a lesion in this hemisphere can partially or totally compromise the function. This means that a patient may have difficulties with comprehension, expression and calculation (CAMBIER, 2005 and SAINBURG, 2006).

The right hemisphere is primarily concerned with spatial organisation, non-verbal ideation (musical activities), the personalisation of features and understanding simple language, such as short sentences and deciphering written language. However, this hemisphere has a low capacity for retaining auditory messages and, above all, has no access to words (CAMBIER, 2004).

The aim of the rehabilitation process is to minimise the impact of the stroke on both the victim and their carer and to optimise the chance of survival. This rehabilitation, which should ideally be as early as possible, reduces mortality, has a positive impact on functionality and reduces the incidence of transfers to long-term care facilities (LEITE, 2005).

The rehabilitation process is part of the therapy and varies from person to person, as with any pathology, since this programme must be stipulated individually, taking into account the particularities of the patient and the surrounding family (LEITE, 2005).

As mentioned above, stroke victims can present different clinical manifestations depending on the area or areas of the brain affected, which is why the Rehabilitation Nurse Specialist must carry out a thorough and precise assessment, evaluating symptoms and the resulting sequelae. This assessment should not neglect the neurological examination, which assesses the different cranial nerves, strength, possible spasticity and balance (CARVALHIDO and PONTES, 2009).

According to PAIS RIBEIRO (2005), the aim of post-stroke rehabilitation is to overcome the disabilities caused by the accident, and there are three possible ways in which individuals with brain damage can recover their lost functional capacities: spontaneous recovery, restitution of function or compensation for lost function.

There is a strong consensus among experts that the most important element in any rehabilitation programme is direct, well-guided and repetitive practice, always bearing in mind that persistence tends to improve technique *(EUROPEAN STROKE ORGANISATION,* 2008).

The ideal duration of rehabilitation has not been definitively clarified, however, there has been an association between increasing the intensity of rehabilitation, especially in the time spent practising ADLs, and improved functional results. Bearing in mind that many immediate complications of stroke are related to immobility, we can consider mobilisation to be a fundamental component of early rehabilitation *(EUROPEAN STROKE INITIATIVE,* 2003).

According to NERI (2001), functional capacity/independence has been defined as the degree of preservation of the individual's ability to carry out basic activities of daily living (BADLs) or self-care and also to develop instrumental activities of daily living (IADLs).

The term activities of daily living appeared in 1954, expressing an individual's independence in everyday activities. In 1963, Katz studied adults and the elderly with chronic illnesses and introduced the term ABVD's, which encompassed activities that allowed these individuals to live in their own environment through self-care actions such as bathing, dressing, hygiene, transference, continence and eating (ITAMI, 2008).

ITAMI (2008) also refers to LAWTON and BRODY (1969) who presented the instrumental activities of daily living (IADLs), which are more complex and include actions such as cooking, tidying the house, telephoning, doing the washing up, going shopping, looking after household finances and taking medication.

At the same time, the term functional assessment was also coined with the aim of objectively measuring an individual's performance in certain areas such as physical, intellectual and emotional health (KAWASAKI, CRUZ E DIOGO, 2004).

Measuring functional independence/dependence makes it possible to monitor the patient's progress in their rehabilitation process, with a view to adjusting therapeutic interventions and checking the speed of gains until a reduction in the acquisition of improvements is established (GREVE, 2007).

The FIM was created in 1984 through the strong commitment of the Academy of Physical Rehabilitation Medicine and the American Congress of Rehabilitation Medicine *(Guide for the uniform data system for medical rehabilitation, 1993).* Its aim was to attempt to standardise concepts and definitions of disability, to obtain a single rehabilitation instrument capable of measuring the degree to which the disabled individual requires third-party care to perform motor and cognitive tasks.

In clinical terms, this instrument makes it possible to determine the severity of the disability, assess and monitor the patient's functional gains and the result obtained, assess the quality of a rehabilitation programme, facilitate the collection of common functional data and compare data on disability and the level of functional disability as a result of rehabilitation treatment (FARIAS and BUCHALLA, 2005).

The MIF Scale measures the areas of self-care, sphincter control, mobility, locomotion, communication and social cognition using scores ranging from one to seven, these values corresponding to the level of dependence on others. Thus, we have **Level 7** - Complete independence (all activities are carried out with help, without modification, safely and in good time); **Level 6 -** Modified independence (the activity carried out requires specialised equipment, a longer than reasonable time to complete or requires safety precautions); **Level 5** - Supervision or preparation (the person needs control, the presence or suggestion of another person, but without physical contact); **Level 4** - help with minimal contact (the person performs 75% or more of the activity); **Level 3** - moderate help (the person performs 50 to 74% of the activity); **Level 2** - maximum help (the person performs less than 50%, but performs at least 25% of the activity); **Level 1** - total help (the person performs less than 25% of the activity) (FARIAS and BUCHALLA, 2005).

CERVEIRA (2011) carried out a study on functional independence in stroke patients, with a sample of 105 individuals, concluding that the variables type of stroke, hemisphere affected and continuity with rehabilitation proved to be very significant in functional recovery. He also concluded that clinical variables have a greater influence on functional independence when tested dimension by dimension.

COELHO (2011) carried out a study on the determinants of the functional capacity of patients after stroke, with a sample of 61 individuals, concluding that the variables with a significant influence on functional capacity were gender, age, type and location of stroke, length of hospital stay, presence of risk factors and rehabilitation programme.

The topic I chose arose from the fact that I provide care at the Alcoitão Rehabilitation Medicine Centre, in the General Adult Rehabilitation service, which has patients with neurological pathologies.

The research questions are specific and include the various aspects that can be studied. They derive directly from the objectives and indicate what the researcher wants to obtain as results (FORTIN, 2009).

In view of the above, two research questions emerged:

+ What is the level of functional independence of the post-stroke patient?

+ To what extent do sociodemographic variables (gender, age, marital status and education) and clinical variables (time of stroke, type of stroke, brain territory affected, acute rehabilitation, repeat stroke, thrombolysis and ongoing rehabilitation programme) influence post-stroke functional independence?

The general objective of the study is to **identify levels of functional independence in post-stroke patients and their correlation with sociodemographic and clinical variables.**

The specific objectives of this study seek to respond to some of the concerns raised by this issue, i.e. they seek in general terms:

Identify sociodemographic variables of post-stroke patients;

-Clinically characterise the post-stroke patient;

-Identify levels of functional independence in post-stroke patients;

-To analyse correlations between sociodemographic and clinical variables and functional independence after stroke;

-Compare levels of functional independence at admission and discharge.

This work is divided into four main points, starting with the materials and methods, followed by the presentation and discussion of the results, and concluding with the conclusion.

In summary, this study will allow us to identify the variables with the greatest impact on functional independence, in order to help define guidelines for the continuous improvement of the care provided.

1.MATERIALS AND METHODS

The process of constructing the study is fundamental for a better understanding and interpretation of the research results. We therefore planned to carry out a descriptive, cross-sectional and analytical-correlational quantitative study.

The type of study is cross-sectional, since the variables in question are studied at a specific point in time. The aim of a cross-sectional or incidence study is to observe, over a period of time, phenomena that influence a group of people with a certain aspect in common (FORTIN, 2009).

We proceeded according to an analytical-correlational logic, with the aim of exploring relationships between variables and their description (FORTIN, 2009). The aim was therefore to describe

Functional Independence after stroke and analyse the influence of sociodemographic and clinical variables on it.

According to FORTIN (2009, p.123): "The link between the frame of reference and the method is ensured by the conceptual or theoretical framework, which defines the nature of the variables to be studied. Establishing this link is particularly important in studies aimed at verifying theoretical propositions, because it is then a question of confirming or disproving hypotheses arising from the theory. The measurement instruments are chosen according to the variables defined in the reference framework."

According to FORTIN (2009), variables are included in the statement of purpose, research questions and hypotheses. They are considered the basic units of the investigation, as well as qualities, properties or characteristics of people, objects or situations that can change or vary over time. The independent variable is the element capable of exerting an effect on another variable being introduced and manipulated in a research context. The dependent variable is the element that suffers the effect, it is the result expected by the researcher (FORTIN, 2009).

To carry out this research, a set of necessary and fundamental variables was considered for statistical treatment. The dependent variable was defined as the functional independence of the post-stroke patient. The independent variables were divided into sociodemographic variables (gender, age, marital status and educational qualifications) and clinical variables (time since stroke, type of stroke, brain territory affected, rehabilitation in the acute phase, repeat stroke, thrombolysis and ongoing rehabilitation programme).

The articulation of the variables studied is represented in the schematic model in Figure 1.

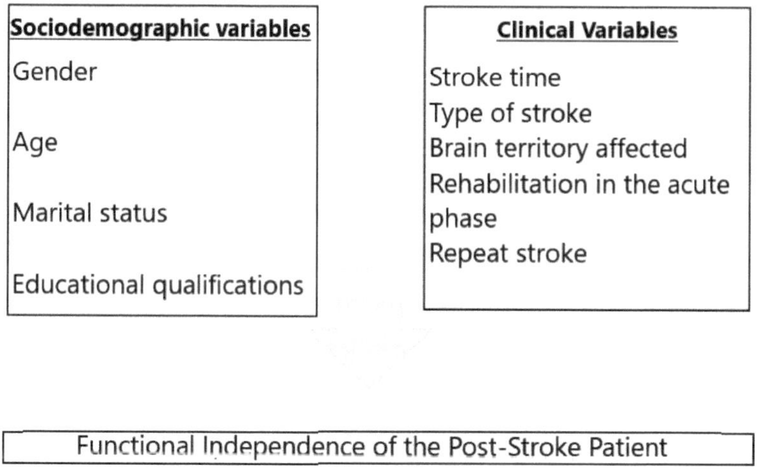

Sociodemographic variables

Gender

Age

Marital status

Educational qualifications

Clinical Variables

Stroke time
Type of stroke
Brain territory affected
Rehabilitation in the acute phase
Repeat stroke

Functional Independence of the Post-Stroke Patient

Figure 1 - Conceptual model of the expected relationship between the variables studied in the empirical research

1.1. PARTICIPANTS

In the context of this research work, we would not be able to study the entire population because it is so large, otherwise it would be very time-consuming, expensive and somewhat difficult to realise.

Given the nature of our study, we used the non-probabilistic convenience sampling method in our research, as it was made up of patients with a diagnosis of stroke admitted to the Rehabilitation Medicine Centre. We are aware that this method is likely to bias some results, as it may not be representative of the target population.

Our sample consisted of 60 participants, 60.0 per cent of whom were male and 40.0 per cent female.

1.2. INSTRUMENTS

According to FORTIN (2009), in order to choose the data collection method, the researcher has to take into account the objectives they want to achieve and thus adapt a method to fulfil their objectives. Only then can the method or instrument for data collection be selected.

Data collection was carried out using a data collection instrument in the form of a questionnaire, which was preceded by a brief introductory note, briefly explaining the purpose of the study, confidentiality and privacy guarantees.

With this in mind, it was decided to collect data by questioning patients individually, using questionnaires and scales, in the following sequence:

-Sociodemographic characterisation questionnaire;

-Clinical characterisation questionnaire;

-Functional Independence Measure Scale (FIM).

Sociodemographic characterisation questionnaire

The questionnaire was constructed on the basis of the research objectives, consultation of the literature and other questionnaires, with the aim of gathering relevant information for sociodemographic characterisation and determining its influence on functional independence after stroke. The questionnaire consists of four questions, three closed and one open. It is subdivided into items about gender, age, marital status and educational qualifications.

Clinical characterisation questionnaire

The questionnaire was constructed on the basis of the research objectives, consultation of the bibliography and other questionnaires, with the aim of gathering relevant information for clinical characterisation and determining its influence on functional independence after stroke. It consists of six questions, five closed and one open. It is subdivided into questions about the time of stroke, type of stroke, territory affected, acute phase rehabilitation, first stroke and thrombolysis.

The last clinical variable, called ongoing rehabilitation programme, is not included in the questionnaire, as all patients admitted to the CMRA are subject to an ongoing rehabilitation programme, which lasts the same length of time as their hospital stay, in which a whole multi-professional team takes part.

Functional Independence Measure Scale - (FIM)

The Functional Independence Measure (FIM) was developed in 1986 by GRANGER *et al.* It is widely used and accepted as a functional assessment measure in the USA and internationally (GRANGER 1986 and BENVEGNU, 2008).

The aim of this instrument was to measure functional capacity using a scale of seven levels representing degrees of functionality, ranging from independence to dependence.

The FIM is an instrument that assesses functional independence, regardless of the physical, communication, functional and emotional sequelae, among others, presented by the patients (BENVEGNU, 2004).

The FIM is mainly used for neurological injuries, such as strokes and spinal cord injuries. This scale provides information through observation of the user's performance and/or information provided by the patient/family/carers/team. Its advantage is that it not only covers motor activities, but also cognitive aspects and communication skills. The MIF Scale is divided into two main domains, motor and cognitive. It has a score that can vary from 18 to 126 points.

Its domains are divided into several dimensions, namely Self-care (6 items with a score of 42/126), Sphincter control (2 items with a score of 14/126), Mobility (3 items 21/126), Locomotion (2 items 14/126), Communication (2 items 14/126), and Social cognition (3items 21/126).

The score for each item varies from one to seven (1 - 7), according to the degree of dependence: 7- complete independence; 6- modified independence; 5- supervision; 4- minimal help (individual performs >=75% of the task); 3- moderate help (individual performs >=50% of the task); 2- maximum help (individual performs >=25% of the task), 1- total help. The total FIM can be divided into four subscores, according to the total score obtained: a) 18 points: complete dependence (total assistance); b) 19 - 60 points: modified dependence (assistance of up to 50% of the task); c) 61 - 103 points: modified dependence (assistance of up to 25% of the task); d) 104 - 126 points: complete / modified independence (2004).

Each item is analysed by the sum of its respective categories. The lower the score, the higher the degree of dependence, and so on.

1.3. PROCEDURES

In view of the study's objectives, the methodology adopted was to administer a questionnaire to hospitalised patients. The scale (MIF) was applied at two different times: at the beginning of hospitalisation and after three months.

A letter was sent to the Centro de Medicina de Reabilitação de Alcoitão (Rehabilitation Medicine Centre of Alcoitão), asking for the questionnaire to be administered, and it was only administered once permission had been granted. This institution was receptive to the study, but the delay in the authorisation process led to a delay in data collection.

The data was collected from 1 September to 30 December 2011, and the average time taken to complete the form was approximately 10 minutes.

The correctly completed questionnaires were numbered and their validity was checked for inclusion in the study, and all those that were incomplete were excluded.

Self-care, the average independence value was 20.03 at the time of admission and 28.30 at the time of discharge, the difference being **statistically significant**, t(59) = -10.482, $p=0.000$.

Sphincter control, the average independence value was 9.90 at the time of admission and 10.65 at the time of discharge, the difference being **statistically significant**, t(59) = -2.922, $p=0.005$.

Mobility, the average independence value was 9.45 at the time of admission and 13.65 at the time of discharge, the difference being **statistically significant**, t(59) = -10.121, $p=0.000$.

Locomotion, the average independence value was 5.43 at the time of admission and 7.77 at the time of discharge, the difference being **statistically significant**, t(59) = -7.581, $p=0.000$.

Communication, the average value of independence is 9.32 at the time of entry and 10.53 at the time of discharge, the difference being **statistically significant**, t(59) = -4.540, $p=0.000$.

In terms of ***social cognition,*** the average independence score was 10.37 at the time of admission and 12.85 at the time of discharge, and the difference was **statistically significant**, $t(59) = 8.273$, $p=0.000$.

In terms of ***social cognition,*** the average independence score was 64.50 at the time of admission and 83.75 at the time of discharge, and the difference was **statistically significant**, $t(59) = 11.264$, $p=0.000$.

DISCUSSION OF RESULTS

Discussion of the results of the sociodemographic variables

The results of the study show that the majority of the participants in the sample are male (60.0%), which supports the opinion of PHIPPS (2003), since according to him, the incidence in males is slightly higher. This opinion is also held by PORTUGAL (2009).

According to PHIPPS (2003), the risk of stroke increases with age, with around 85 per cent occurring in people over the age of 65 and a stroke rarely occurring before the age of 55. According to the data from our study, the most representative age groups are 51-60 and 61-70 years old, which leads us to easily conclude that this pathology is increasingly affecting young people, and may be related to the sedentary lifestyle that has been increasing in our society. The results of our study are in line with those obtained by PORTUGAL (2009), since according to the 2005/2006 national health survey, there were around 1,629 Portuguese stroke victims between the ages of 45 and 54.

Focusing on the marital status variable, we found that the majority of the participants in the sample were married (61.0%), followed by divorced (17.0%) and widowed (15.0%). These figures are in line with the data collected on 31 December 2003, when it was estimated that around 49.50% of the resident population in Portugal was married (LEITE, 2005).

According to MARQUES et al. (2006), a low level of education can make it difficult to realise the need for lifelong health care, adhere to treatment and maintain healthy lifestyles. With regard to educational qualifications, this study found that 42.0% had secondary education, 40.0% had basic education and only 15.0% had a degree **Discussion of the results of the clinical variables**

The results of the study show that most of the participants in the sample had their stroke less than 2 months previously (63.3 per cent), taking into account the date of admission.

With regard to the type of stroke, it should be noted that according to the data obtained, 81.7% of the participants in the sample were victims of an ischaemic stroke, which reinforces the idea of FERRO (2006), insofar as he believes that around 85% of strokes are ischaemic and 15% haemorrhagic.

Taking into account the brain territory affected, it can be noted that 55% of the participants in the sample had a stroke in the left hemisphere and only 43.3% in the right hemisphere. These figures are in line with the opinion of VENTURA (2002), since according to a study entitled "Functional Independence in Stroke Patients: Influence of the Hemisphere Affected", 51% of the sample had a left hemisphere lesion and 49% had a right hemisphere lesion.

With regard to rehabilitation in the acute phase, 85% of the participants had access to it, which demonstrates the importance of the Rehabilitation Course, since it was not possible to achieve these figures with the specialists who existed before the speciality in this area was reopened, since the vast majority of them went on to hold senior positions. In view of the above, it can be said that it is now possible to put into practice the opinion of LEITE (2005), who supports the idea that rehabilitation should be carried out as early as possible.

Discussion of the results of the hypothesis testing variables

GRAY *et al* (2007) refer to GLADER *et al* (2003) and KRAPAL *et al* (2005) to prove that the results obtained in post-stroke recovery are less significant in females when compared to males. In our study, it was found that gender did not significantly influence the functional independence of the participants. This result is in line with the opinion of PORTUGAL (2009), who found that there was no statistically significant difference in the evolution of functional independence according to gender.

HAASE and LACERDA (2004) state that the possibility of functional recovery is inversely proportional to age, i.e. the younger the individual, the greater the possibility of recovery, due to cerebral neuroplasticity. However, BAGG, POMBO and HOPMAN (2002), after analysing fourteen studies, concluded that the age factor does not contribute significantly to the functional outcome, which is in line with the results of our study, in that no significant influence was found between age and the participants' functional independence.

In our study, marital status did not significantly influence the participants' functional independence, but we did find statistically significant differences in the self-care dimension.

Contrary to what might have been predicted, educational qualifications did not significantly influence the functional independence of the participants, which allows us to conclude that the teachings were always appropriate to each person's ability to understand and assimilate.

The length of time since the stroke did not significantly influence the participants' functional independence, since there was only a significant difference in terms of self-care, sphincters and locomotion. The aforementioned data can be easily justified, as 91.7 per cent underwent rehabilitation in the acute phase. It can therefore be concluded that the waiting time that sometimes limits patients' access to a specialised centre is, in most cases, being compensated for with rehabilitation programmes.

According to CHAE *et al* (1996; Silva 2010) haemorrhagic strokes are generally more serious than ischaemic strokes, and this opinion is shared by ROCHA (2008), insofar as he assumes that haemorrhagic strokes are the worst in terms of prognosis. Despite this, we found no statistically significant differences between the type of stroke and the participants' functional independence.

VOOS and VALE (2007) carried out a study to assess whether left hemisphere lesions cause different motor impairments to right hemisphere lesions. It is known that there is greater impairment of voluntary movement in left hemispheric lesions, while there is a notable loss of spatial attention and postural control when the lesion occurs in the right hemisphere. According to VENTURA (2002), the "social cognition" dimension is not statistically significant, and it cannot be inferred that patients with left-sided lesions show greater functional evolution than those with right-sided lesions. However, they are in harmony with regard to the "mobility" dimension. In our study, the territory affected did not significantly influence the participants' functional independence.

According to TEIXEIRA-SALMELA *et al* (2003), rehabilitation should begin as early as possible, as it can reduce the number of patients who become dependent after a stroke. If active rehabilitation is not possible, passive rehabilitation should be carried out, minimising the risks resulting from immobility, as these are complications that can reduce the individual's potential for recovery. This idea is also defended by DUNCAN (2005), who believes that rehabilitation should be early and intensive in order to obtain functional benefits, and that as soon as the patient's clinical situation stabilises, efforts should be made to ensure their functional recovery. In our study, it was concluded that rehabilitation in the acute phase of the participants in the sample significantly influenced their functional independence, more specifically in terms of self-care, mobility and locomotion, in line with the opinion of the aforementioned authors.

In a study carried out by ABREU (2009) at the Stroke Unit of the Cova da Beira Hospital Centre, it was found that patients who underwent thrombolysis had a very positive response to the treatment. However, not all authors support the same idea, as Teixeira (2004) found that thrombolytic treatment was not effective and increased the risk of intracranial haemorrhage. In our study, we found no statistically significant differences between thrombolysis and functional independence.

In a study carried out by BENVEGNU *et al* (2008), which assessed the evolution of functional independence in individuals with strokes in carrying out activities of daily living who underwent phytotherapeutic treatment during the hospital phase, it was concluded that there was a significant difference between the initial and final scores, with the items "self-care", "locomotion" and "communication" showing the greatest evolution. Our study concluded that the ongoing rehabilitation programme had a statistically significant influence on all dimensions of functional independence.

CONCLUSION

This study aimed to achieve the two objectives mentioned in the introduction. The sociodemographic and clinical characteristics of the sample were described. In addition, a level of functional independence was described and a set of variables that could influence patients' functional independence was identified. In this way, we believe we have made a contribution to the knowledge of statistically significant associative relationships in the field of functional independence.

With regard to **sociodemographic** characterisation, we can point out that 60 participants took part in the study, 60.0% of whom were male. With regard to marital status, 61.0% were married and 17.0% divorced. With regard to educational qualifications, 41.7% had secondary education, 40.0% had basic education and only 15.0% had a degree.

With regard to **clinical characterisation**, we can say that the majority of participants had their stroke less than 2 months previously (63.3%), a fairly high percentage had an ischaemic stroke (81.7%), and just over half affected the left hemisphere (55.0%). We can also point out that 85% of the participants underwent rehabilitation in the acute phase, for almost all of them this was their first stroke (91.7%) and approximately a third (31.7%) of the participants underwent thrombolysis.

With regard to characterising **levels of functional independence**, we can point out that there was an increase in functional independence in all dimensions of the Functional Independence Measurement Scale (FIM) when comparing the time of entry with the time of discharge.

With regard to the **hypotheses studied**, we can emphasise that we accept the following hypotheses and reject the others (Hi, H2, H4, He, H7 and H9):

- **H3** - Marital status did not significantly influence the participants' functional independence, but we did find statistically significant differences in the self-care dimension;
- **H5** - The duration of the stroke did not significantly influence the functional independence of the participants, but we did find statistically significant differences in the self-care, sphincter and locomotion dimensions;
- **He** - Rehabilitation in the acute phase of the participants in the sample significantly influenced their functional independence, finding statistically significant differences in the self-care, locomotion and mobility dimensions;
- **H10** - The ongoing rehabilitation programme had a statistically significant influence on functional independence.

In view of the above, we can conclude that clinical variables have a greater influence on functional independence when tested dimension by dimension, namely the length of time since the stroke, rehabilitation in the acute phase and the ongoing rehabilitation programme.

STUDY LIMITATIONS AND SUGGESTIONS

As far as the sample is concerned, we initially wanted to try to gather as many people as possible and ensure that they were representative of the general population. The questionnaire and information on how to fill it in was delivered to the Alcoitão Rehabilitation Medicine centre, so we believe that our sample should be made up of a larger number of patients. However, time limitations meant that we were unable to obtain a large sample, preventing us from making any generalisations.

As we are aware of our limitations, we suggest further research in this area with a larger number of participants, so that its representativeness can be generalised to the population in general.

We should also emphasise the importance of developing future research that integrates other independent variables from a psychological and clinical context.

We conclude by emphasising that there is much to be done and researched in the field of functional independence, but we can only congratulate ourselves on the results obtained, as we believe we have contributed to understanding this complex phenomenon that is the functional independence of post-stroke patients.

BIBLIOGRAPHICAL REFERENCES

- ABREU, S ; DAMASCENO A. - Stroke Help: online carer's manual. Journal of the Portuguese Society of Physical Medicine and Rehabilitation. Year 17, Vol. 17, No. 1 (January-February, 2009).
- ANDRÉ, C. - **Stroke Manual**. Rio de Janeiro: Revinter, 1999.
- BAGG, S. ; POMBO, A. P. ; HOPMAN, W. - Effect of age on functional outcomes after stroke rehabilitation. Stroke. 33 (2002), p. 179-185
- BENVEGNU, A. B. ; Gomes L. A. ; SOUZA, C. T. - Evaluation of the measure of functional independence of individuals with sequelae of cerebrovascular accident (CVA). Journal Ciência & Saúde. Porto Alegre. Vol. 1, n° 2 (July/December, 2008), p. 71-77.
- CAMBIER, Jean; MASSON, Maurice; DEHEN, Henri - **Neurology**. 11ª ed. Rio de Janeiro: Guanabara Koogan, 2005. ISBN 85-2771066-8.
- CARMONA, J. - **Hypertension is the main cause of strokes** [Online]. 2004 [Consulted on 11 January 2011]. Available from WWW: < URL:http:www. spavc. org/imgs/content/article 42/sp5. pdf>.
- CARVALHIDO, Teresa; PONTES, Manuela - Home-based rehabilitation for people who have suffered a stroke. Journal of the Faculty of Health Sciences of Porto. ISSN 1646-0480. N°6 (2009), p. 140-150.

- CERVEIRA, Joel Andrade - Functional independence in stroke patients: sociodemographic and clinical determinants. Master's degree in rehabilitation nursing. Work supervised by Prof Helena Moreira. June 2011.
- CHAVES, Marcia Loureiro F. - Routines in Neurology and Neurosurgery. Porto Alegre: artemed, 2008, p. 97-127.
- COELHO, Rosa Maria Alves - Determinants of Functional Capacity of Patients after Stroke - Volume II. Master's degree in rehabilitation nursing. Work carried out under the supervision of Professor Carlos Albuquerque. December 2011.
- DUNCAN, P. [et al.] - Management of adult stroke rehabilitation care: a clinical practice guideline. Stroke [Online]. Vol. 36, n° 9 (September 2005), 100-043.
  [Consulted 27 Feb. 2012]. Available at WWW:<URL: http://stroke.ahajournals.org/content/36Z9/e100.full.pdf>.
- EUROPEAN STROKE INICIATIVE - **Ischaemic stroke: prophylaxis and treatment**. Germany: EUSI, 2003.
- EUROPEAN STROKE INITIATIVE - Cerebrovascular disease: recommendations for stroke management. Cerebrovascular Diseases [Online]. N° 16 (2003), p. 311-337 [Consulted 27 Feb. 2012]. Available at WWW: <URL http://www.esostroke.org/pdf/EUSI2003_Cerebrovasc_Dis.pdf>.
- EUROPEAN STROKE ORGANISATION - **Recommendations for the treatment of ischaemic stroke 2008** [Online]. Heidelberg, 2008. [Consulted 23 Feb 2012]. Available at WWW:<URL: http://www.eso-strok.org/pdf/ESO08_Guidelines_Portuguese.pdf>.
- FARIAS, Norma; BUCHALLA, Cassia Maria - The International

Classification of Functioning, Disability and Health of the World Health Organisation: Uses and perspectives. Revista brasileira de epidemiologia. [Online]. Vol. 8, n°2 (2005), p.187192 [cited on 12 March 2012]. Available at <http//www.scielo.br/pdf/rbepid/v8n2/11.pdf>

- FERRO, José Maria - Epidemiology, risk factors and primary prevention of stroke. Pathos. Lisbon. N° 7 (July/August 2000), p.7-17.
- FERRO, José Maria - 21st century stroke prevention. Pathos. Lisbon. N° 7, (July/August 2000), p. 30-36.
- FERRO, José Maria; PIMENTEL, J. - **Neurology: principles, diagnosis and treatment**. Lisbon: Lidel, 2006.
- FORTIN, Marie Fabienne - **Fundamentals and stages of the research process**. Lisbon: Lusodidacta, 2009. ISBN 9789898075185.
- GONÇALVES, Cátia Susana Almeida -Functional dependence of the elderly after stroke. Master's degree in rehabilitation nursing. Work carried out under the supervision of Professor Rosa Martins. Viseu ESSV May 2011.
- GRANGER C. V. ; Hamilton B. B.; Keith R. A. - **Advances in functional assessment for medical rehabilitation: topics in geriatric rehabilitation**, Rockville: Aspen, 1986.
- GRAY, J. [et al.] - Sex differences in quality of life in stroke survivors: data from the tinzaparin in acute ischaemic stroke trial (TAIST). Stroke [Online]. Vol. 38, n°11 (November 2007), p. 2960-2964. [Consulted 23 Feb. 2012]. Available at WWW:<URL: http://stroke.ahajournals.org/content/38/11/2960.full.pdf>.

- GREVE, J. - Treatise on rehabilitation medicine. São Paulo. Roca, 2007.
- HAASE, Vítor Geraldi; LACERDA, Shirley Silva. - Neuroplasticity, interindividual variation and functional recovery in neuropsychology. SBP Topics in Psychology. Ribeirão Preto. ISSN 1413-389X. Vol. 12, n° 1 (January/February 2004), p. 28-42.
- ITAMI, L.T. - **External causes and their impact on functional independence in adults with fractures**. University of São Paulo: EEUSP, 2008.
- KAWASAKI, K.; CRUZ, K.C.T.; DIOGO, M.J.D. - The use of the measure of functional independence in the elderly: a bibliographical review. Rehabilitation Medicine. 2004 p.57-60.
- KOIZUMI, Maria Sumie; DICCINI, Solange - Enfermagem em Neurociência: São Paulo: Athneu, 2006, p.329-335.
- MARÔCO, João - **Statistical analysis with PASW: ex SPSS**. Pêro Pinheiro: Report Number, 2010.
- MARÔCO, João - **Statistical analysis: using SPSS**. Lisbon: Silabo, 2007.
- MARQUES, Sueli; RODRIGUES, Rosalina Aparecida Partezani; KUSUMOTA, Lucina - The elderly after stroke: changes in family relationships. Revista Latino-Americana de Enfermagem [Online]. Vol. 14, n°3 (May/June 2006), p. 1-8. [Consult. 12 Dec. 2011]. Available at WWW:<URL:www.eerp.usp.br/rlae>.
- NERI, A. L. - **Development and ageing**. Campinas: Papirus, 2001.
- NOGUEIRA, J. M. Abreu [et al.] - **Framework for stroke rehabilitation units: long-term health care and social support** [Online]. Lisbon, July 2007. [Consult. 28 Feb. 2012]. Available at WWW:< URL:http://www.umcci.min

saude.pt/SiteCollectionDocuments/UnidadesReabilitacaodeAV CfinalR ESUMOEX ECUTIVO.pdf>.

- PAIS-RIBEIRO, Jose Luis - Introduction to health psychology. Coimbra: quarteto 2005. ISBN 989-558-045-2.
- PESTANA, M. H.; GAGEIRO, J. N. - **Data analysis for social sciences**. 4ª ed. Lisbon: Edições Sílabo, 2005.
- PHIPPS, W. J., Sands, J. K., Marek, J. F. - **Medical-surgical nursing**: **concepts and clinical practice**. 6ª ed. Loures: Lusociência, 2003. ISBN 972-838365-7.
- POLIT, Denise F.; BEEK, Cheryl Tatamo - Fundamentals of Nursing Research. 7th ed. Porto Alegre: Artemed, 2011.
- PORTUGAL. Directorate-General for Health - Risk of dying in Portugal: National health survey. 2005/2006. Lisbon: DGS, 2009.
- PORTUGAL. National Statistics Institute - Risk of dying in Portugal. Lisbon: DGS, 2000.
- PORTUGAL. Ministry of Health - High Commission for Health. National Coordination for Cardiovascular Diseases - **Clinical recommendations for acute myocardial infarction and stroke**. Lisbon: ACS 2007. ISBN 978-989-951462-1. [Consulted 2 Feb 2011]. Available at WWW:<URL:http://www.acs.min-saude.pt>.
- PORTUGAL. Ministry of Health. General Directorate of Health. Directorate of Planning Services - **Stroke Units: recommendations for their development**. Lisbon: D G S, 2001. ISBN 972-942597-3.
- M. ; Miyazaki M. H. ; JUCÁ, S. S. H. Validation of the Brazilian version of the functional independence measure. Ata Fisiátrica.

Vol. 11, n. 2, (March/April 2004), p. 72-76.

- ROCHA, S. I. M. - **Acute cerebrovascular disease: evaluation of a thrombolysis protocol: Stroke Unit, Cova da Beira Hospital Centre, EPE.** Covilhã: Faculty of Health Sciences, 2008.

  Integrated master's thesis in medicine, presented to the Faculty of Sciences of the UBI, Covilhã.

- SAINBURG, Robert L. [et al.] - Does motor lateralisation have implications for stroke rehabilitation? Journal of Rehabilitation Development. Vol. 43, n° 3, (may/june 2006), p. 311-322.

- SILVA, E. J. A. - **Rehabilitation after stroke**. Porto: Faculty of Medicine of Porto, 2010. Integrated Master's Dissertation in Medicine, area: Community Medicine.

- SULLIVAN, Susan B.; SCHMITZ, Thomas J. - Physiotherapy, assessment and treatment -2ª Edition São Paulo, Editora Manole, 1993.

- TEIXEIRA, Ricardo; SILVA, Leonardo; FERREIRA, Valerio - Thrombolytic treatment in ischaemic stroke - Revista Neurociencias. São Paulo. ISSN 0104-3579, Vol. 12, n°1 (2004), p. 517.

- TEIXEIRA-SALMELA, L.F.. et al. - Weight training and aerobic conditioning in the functional performance of chronic hemiplegics. Acta Fisiátrica. Vol.10, N° 2, 2003, p.54-60.

- VENTURA, Maria Clara Amado Apóstolo - Functional independence in stroke patients: influence of the affected hemisphere. In: Referência. - Coimbra. - ISSN 0874-0283. - No.

9 (November 2002), p. 31-40.

- VOOS, M.C.; VALLE, Ribeiro do - Functional asymmetries in patients with hemiparesis: a literature review. Brazilian Journal of Physiotherapy. Vol.14 N° 1, 2007, p.79-87.

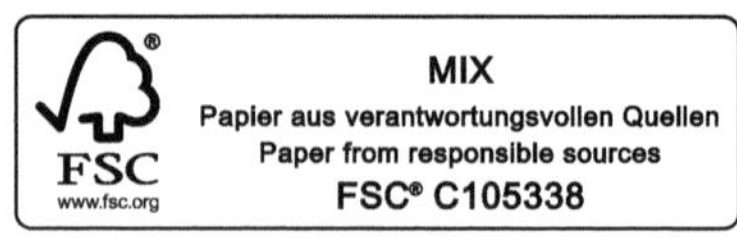

Printed by Books on Demand GmbH, Norderstedt / Germany